I0091397

Rizwana Ansari

Current Intrapartum Care Practices in India

Rizwana Ansari

Current Intrapartum Care Practices in India

Opinion and Beliefs on Routine versus Evidence based Practice during Childbirth

VDM Verlag Dr. Müller

Imprint

Bibliographic information by the German National Library: The German National Library lists this publication at the German National Bibliography; detailed bibliographic information is available on the Internet at http://dnb.d-nb.de.

Any brand names and product names mentioned in this book are subject to trademark, brand or patent protection and are trademarks or registered trademarks of their respective holders. The use of brand names, product names, common names, trade names, product descriptions etc. even without a particular marking in this works is in no way to be construed to mean that such names may be regarded as unrestricted in respect of trademark and brand protection legislation and could thus be used by anyone.

Cover image: www.purestockx.com

Publisher:
VDM Verlag Dr. Müller Aktiengesellschaft & Co. KG , Dudweiler Landstr. 125 a, 66123 Saarbrücken, Germany,
Phone +49 681 9100-698, Fax +49 681 9100-988,
Email: info@vdm-verlag.de

Zugl.: Durham, University of New Hampshire, September 2006

Copyright © 2008 VDM Verlag Dr. Müller Aktiengesellschaft & Co. KG and licensors
All rights reserved. Saarbrücken 2008

Produced in USA and UK by:
Lightning Source Inc., La Vergne, Tennessee, USA
Lightning Source UK Ltd., Milton Keynes, UK
BookSurge LLC, 5341 Dorchester Road, Suite 16, North Charleston, SC 29418, USA

ISBN: 978-3-639-01451-8

DEDICATION

This thesis is dedicated to my parents for providing me their enduring strength,

courage, support, and blessings.

1

ACKNOWLEDGEMENTS

I would like to acknowledge my thesis committee members, Dr. Gene Harkless, Dr. Lynette Ament, and Martha D. Leighton, for their immense guidance and support during the development of this research work.

I would like to extend my deepest gratitude to Chair of my committee Dr. Gene Harkless, for her great guidance and support. She has inspired me to enter this graduate program and pursue my degree from UNH. She has always been a tremendous resource to me, without her expertise in nursing research this work would have never been a success. I met Dr. Gene Harkless in India prior coming to United States. I will always remember the time when I met her and explored all the opportunities for pursuing an advanced degree in nursing. She introduced me to the real world of Evidence-Based Nursing Practice. Her expertise and tremendous knowledge and skill in nursing research have brought a remarkable starting point in my professional life. I am highly indebted for her astute guidance in designing my research and manuscript preparation.

I must thank Dr. Lynette Ament who has always provided a great support as a Chair of the Department and second reader of my thesis committee to get this work finished on time. She has shown a great interest in my research work. She has always helped me providing excellent literature to support the writing of this thesis.

My special thank goes to Martha Leighton who has taken out time from her busy schedule to go through my thesis reading and guiding me through the process of its further development.

I must thank all the faculty members and administrative members of the Nursing Department for their wonderful help and support.

Last but not least, I must thank my family, friends, colleagues, and many individuals who have been a source of encouragement in making this program a great success.

3

TABLE OF CONTENTS

DEDICATION..1

ACKNOWLEDGEMENTS..2

LIST OF TABLES..6

CHAPTER   PAGE

I. INTRODUCTION..8

II. REVIEW OF LITERATURE..13

    Evidence-Based Childbirth Care..13

    Intrapartum Care Practices..15

        Episiotomy...15

        Labor Induction..17

        Birthing Position...19

        Continuous Support during Labor..20

        Fundal Pressure...22

        Labor Pain Management...24

        Communication of Information & Instructions.................................26

    Difference in Care Providers' Opinions and Practices.......................27

III. METHODOLOGY..29

    Sample...30

    Instruments..30

    Procedure..30

    Human Subjects..31

IV. DATA ANALYSIS..32

    Sample Demographics..32

    Reported Intrapartum Care Practices...34

    Comparison of Findings with WHO Guidelines on Intrapartum Care practices..39

Difference in the Intrapartum Care Practices between Doctors and Nurse-Midwives...41

Difference in the Intrapartum Care Practices of Professionals in Government and Non-Government Hospitals..43

Responses to Open-ended Questions...45

V. DISCUSSION OF THE FINDINGS...47

Limitations..51

Conclusion...51

Implications for Future Practice...52

Implications for Future Research...52

Summary 53

REFERENCES 54

APPENDICES..61

APPENDIX A. SURVEY QUESTIONNAIRE...62

APPENDIX B. INFORMED CONSENT..69

APPENDIX C. UNH INSTITUTIONAL REVIEW BOARD APPROVAL.............71

LIST OF TABLES

TITLE   **PAGE**

Table 1. Demographics..33

Table 2. Frequency Distribution for Normal Birth Attending Personnel........33

Table 3. Frequency Distribution for Written Clinical Practice Policy............33

Table 4. Frequency Distribution for Opinion towards Episiotomy...............34

Table 5. Frequency Distribution for Episiotomy Practice.........................34

Table 6. Frequency Distribution for Considering Women's Preference for

Episiotomy..35

Table 7. Frequency Distribution for Discomfort and Vulval-Hematoma.........35

Table 8. Frequency Distribution for Labor Pain Relief Methods..................36

Table 9. Mean Percentage for Women Receiving Pain Relief Measures.......36

Table10. Frequency Distribution for Birthing Position..............................37

Table 11. Frequency Distribution for Labor Induction..............................37

Table 12. Mean Percentage for Low Risk Women Receiving
Labor Induction...38

Table 13. Frequency Distribution for Practicing Fundal Pressure................38

Table 14. Frequency Distribution for Routine Information..........................38

Table 15. Frequency Distribution for Support Person..............................39

Table 16. Comparison of study findings with WHO guidelines....................40

Table 17. Mean Opinions toward Episiotomy Practice in Professional
Group..41

Table 18. Mean Practice of Episiotomy, Fundal Pressure, & Birthing
Position in Professional Group..42

Table 19. Mean Perception of Discomfort and Vulval-hematoma in
Professional Group..42

Table 20. Mean Preference of Episiotomy Practice in Hospital Group..........43

Table 21. Mean Practice of Episiotomy, Fundal Pressure, & Birthing
    Position in Hospital Group...44

CHAPTER I

INTRODUCTION

Maternal mortality rate in developing countries are staggering, with over 529,000 women in developing countries dying every year due to pregnancy related causes, or are caused by any interventions, omissions, or inappropriate treatment related to pregnancy and childbirth care (WHO, 2005). This reflects a global ratio of 400 maternal deaths per 100,000 live births. India alone accounts for a quarter of these deaths and has the third highest maternal mortality rate among South Asian countries (Rodrigues & Thapar, 2005). According to a report from the Government of India (2001-2002) in 2000 maternal mortality rate in India was 407 per 100,000 live births. This rate remained the same through 2004 (Surg, 2005).

Hence, reducing maternal mortality and morbidity in India is one of the major goals of the Government of India. In India, over 90% of women become mothers and the majority of them deliver without skilled assistance during delivery. This translates to approximately 30 million women in India who experience pregnancy every year, and 27 million who give birth to live infants (Bakshi, 2006). Of these, 136,000 maternal deaths occur every year due to childbirth complications, most of which are believed to be preventable. Even with the high mortality rate in India, the specific pregnancy and childbirth related factors directly responsible for the maternal deaths somewhat invisible (Bakshi, 2006). Overall, the major causes responsible for most of the maternal deaths are due to poor quality care resulting in hemorrhage (25%), puerperal infection (15%), pre-existing disease conditions such as anemia or HIV/AIDS (20%), and other labor and delivery complications (8%) (WHO, 2005). A study of health care professionals reported their belief that lack of skilled birth attendants and shortage of primary medical care

8

centers along with abundant ignorant behavior among woman's family members have contributed to India having one of the worst on maternal mortality rates (Rodrigues & Thapar, 2005). A survey of 7635 women who had experienced childbirth demonstrated that in India basic childbirth care was perceived as inaccessible and of poor quality (Shariff & Singh, 2002).

Care provided during childbirth has significant relevance to the birth outcomes, as routine harmful practices may contribute to childbirth complications interfering with the women's health and autonomy (Wick, Mikki, Giacaman, & Abdul-Rahim, 2005). United Nations Children's Fund (UNICEF) India (2004) reported that technical incompetence and negligence among health care providers are often factors responsible for maternal deaths along with the ineffective health care system, uninformed care providers, and social attitudes that do not promote a safe delivery environment. Health care provider behaviors are influenced by system failures and limited knowledge which then influences the clinician's decision making during childbirth. Overall, the majority of childbirth decisions are still made entirely on the basis of professionals' personal belief, tradition, anecdote, and clinical observations, rather than the evidence based research findings (Volmink, Murphy, & Woldehanna, 2002). It is reported by WHO that health care practices which are inconsistent with evidence-based practice may cause harm to the patients (Smith, Gulmezoglu, & Garner, 2004). For example, a systematic review evaluating the common practice of performing episiotomies suggests that women who receive episiotomy as a routine care have worse outcomes than those who avoid receiving this intervention (Carroli, & Belizan, 2000).

How do practices such as episiotomies become routine and expected during childbirth? Kitzinger, et al., (2006) discusses at length the relationship of birth as a normal process in the context of increasing technological interventions. These authors describe that care-givers are fraught with anxiety about the risks and potential childbirth complications that is due to the medicalization of normal childbirth. Therefore, care providers intervene "just in case" with medical procedures such as labor induction and

9

augmentation, electronic fetal monitoring, narcotics and epidurals for labor pain, as well as other medical interventions, including episiotomies. These authors further suggest that this is how unnecessary medical interventions merge into routine care practices. To break this circle of anxiety and intervention, evidence-based practice may provide clear guidance about when and when not to use technological interventions.

Although evidence-based practice is not unknown in developing countries such as India, the reality of actual childbirth practice is often that is not based on scientific evidence. A recent study by Qian, Smith, Liang, Liang, & Garner (2006) attempted to introduce evidence-based intrapartum care practices in four Chinese hospitals but was unsuccessful. Despite the emphasis on improving maternal health care in India, no studies were found by this researcher that described routine intrapartum care practices from the point of the provider in either public or private institutions.

The standards for safe and effective childbirth care practices have been very well defined by WHO (1999).These standards were developed from the best available evidence and are aimed at improving maternal and fetal outcomes. Yet a significant gap exists between current practice and evidence-informed care in India. Stetler (1999, p.15) stated that "in contrast to routine, mindless, and habitual clinical practice, evidence-based care is an approach that de-emphasizes ritual, isolated and unsystematic clinical experiences, and ungrounded opinion and traditions as a basis for safe and effective quality care practice". Both developed and developing countries are challenged to use evidence to provide safe, high quality care (Wick, et al., 2005). To use the limited resources wisely, it is essential for care providers to base their practice on scientific evidence. The question of how have maternity care providers in India incorporated the WHO guidelines emerges. Also, the practice of safe and effective maternity care as well as the "cooperation, agreement, and divergence in knowledge and opinions" among the care team members rises (Reime et al., 2004, p.1388). Therefore it is also important to understand the differences in opinions and care practices between care providers, including nurse-midwives and doctors. As evidence shows that in developing countries as diverse as Malaysia, Sri Lanka and Tunisia, investments in training, recruiting and retaining midwives have significantly reduced maternal death rates (UNFPA, 2006). It is believed that urgent support to midwives worldwide would save the lives of 5 million women and prevent 80 million pregnancy and childbirth related maternal morbidity by the year 2015 (UNFPA, 2006).

Out of the Oxford Publication Effective Care in Pregnancy and Childbirth (1989), which formed the foundation for the Cochrane Database for Systematic Reviews, an evidence-based approach to obstetrics has evolved to provide best practice information on childbirth (Volmink, et al., 2002). Access to this information is difficult in low resourced countries. Hence, the WHO Reproductive Health Library project was initiated in 1997 in order to provide high quality, evidence-based information to midwives and doctors in developing countries (Gulmezoglu, & Villar, 2002).The motivation to introduce this project was to help health care providers change their routine but harmful childbirth care practice (Gulmezoglu, & Villar, 2002).

Therefore, in order to improve maternal health outcomes and reduce the maternal mortality rate during childbirth, developing countries need best practice information to improve care. However, it is unclear how much knowledge has been disseminated and what maternity care providers have done with this knowledge if it has been transmitted. To begin to answer this question, this author believed that it is useful to ask maternity care providers what they know and what they do regarding the best practice recommendations put forward by WHO (WHO,1999). The WHO recommendations can be used as a standard to compare the self report of maternity care providers in India. Comparing current care practice with recommended evidence-based practice may help to improve maternal care by highlighting areas in need of improvement. The concept of evidence-based care may or may not be a new concept among the maternity care providers in India. Evidence-based practice standards may compete with personal attitude, habits, and practice rituals which may still be very powerful determinants of childbirth practice. Therefore, the first step in achieving

11

evidence-based care is to understand the opinions of professionals towards evidence-based obstetrical care standard and to examine self-reports of how these professionals practice. This information then can be compared to the WHO best practice maternal care policies. Hence, this study proposes to survey maternity care providers (nurse-midwives and doctors) as to their opinions and current practices during intrapartum care management. The research questions are as follows:

Research Questions:-

1. What are the intrapartum care practices as reported by the respondents? including episiotomy, labor induction, childbirth support, labor pain management, fundal pressure, birthing position, and communication of information and instructions to women during intrapartum phase.

2. How do these reported intrapartum care practices compare with the WHO practice guidelines?

3. What are the differences in the intrapartum care practices between doctors and nurse-midwives?

4. What are the differences in the intrapartum care practices between government and non-government hospitals?

It is difficult and beyond the scope of this research to directly quantify and link the care practices including, episiotomy, labor induction, birthing position, childbirth support, fundal pressure, and communication of information and instructions, with the severe consequences of maternal mortality. The following view of literature describes these care practices and how they may be linked to maternal morbidity, but it is beyond the scope of this review of literature to directly quantify the harmful effects of poor maternal care practices on maternal mortality and morbidity.

12

CHAPTER II

REVIEW OF LITERATURE

The purpose of this literature review is to identify scientific research that addresses evidence-based intrapartum care management of childbirth process. This chapter initially presents an overview of the significance of evidence-based childbirth care, followed by a discussion of empirical significance of the seven elements of intrapartum care, including episiotomy, labor induction, labor pain management, childbirth support, birthing position, fundal pressure, and communication of information and instructions to mothers during labor and delivery. And last, this chapter presents a brief discussion of literature on the difference in care practices between nurse-midwives and doctors.

Evidence-Based Childbirth Care

Evidence-based care has been described as " the judicious use of the best evidence available so that the clinician and the patient arrive at the best decision taking into account the needs and values of the individual patient" (Sackette, Rosenberg, Gray, Haynes, & Richardson, 1996, p. 312). Thus, evidence-based practice requires three competencies. The first is the care providers' ability to use correct information required under particular situation. The second requires the clinicians consider the needs and values of individuals receiving care. The third requires that the care providers take into account patient choices in the particular situation (McCandlish, 2001). According to McCandlish, the application of these principles of evidence-based practices might help to foster best care for women during childbirth.

In 1979, Dr. Cochrane's remark about "obstetrics as the medical specialty with the worst record of basing its practice on sound research" (Dickersin & Manheimer, 1998, p. 317), started an international effort to find, evaluate, and summarize the findings from the best studies of the effectiveness of methods used to care for pregnant women (Rooks, 1999). As a result of this effort the Cochrane and WHO Reproductive Health library provides comprehensive recommendations for care during normal childbirth (World Health Organization, 2005). The Cochrane Collaboration produces systematic reviews that summarize and synthesize the research findings from randomized controlled trials to provide current evidence on the safety and efficacy of a wide range of medical care practices in different medical care specialties. Using this knowledge, the goal of WHO Reproductive Health Library (RHL) is to change the practice behaviors of care providers while providing the most up to date reliable sources of evidence-based childbirth care (Gulmezoglu & Villar, 2002). A book entitled *Care in Normal Birth: A Practical Guide*, published by WHO in 1999, is one of the important resource on evidence-based maternity care (World Health Organization, 1999). The book is based on systematic reviews of Cochrane Collaboration. Based on the WHO guidelines, programs like Maternal and Neonatal Health (MNH) have been started in regions of Africa, Asia, Latin America, and the Caribbean to develop groups of regional experts in maternal and newborn care. The MNH program which was initiated between 2000 and 2003, proved to be helpful in strengthening the clinical practice, training, and leadership skills of maternity care providers in South Asia (Blouse, Kinzie, Sanghvi, & Hines, 2004). However, it is unclear how influential this program has been with maternity care providers in India.

National maternal health programs in India such as Reproductive and Child Health and Maternal and Perinatal Death Inquiries (MAPEDI) have been initiated in collaboration with UNICEF to establish the base for evidence-based health care planning in basic health care systems (Bakshi, 2006). These programs are designed to identify the contributing biological, social, and health system factors for maternal deaths. However, it has always been a challenge for the Indian health care system to identify these factors as

14

they are usually under-reported by the care providers, hence, the health system fails to record all maternal deaths accurately (Bakshi, 2006). Despite implementing a number of Maternal Health Care Programs and bringing awareness to improve maternal health among care providers, the overall numbers of women receiving optimum obstetric care are still far below the target of the Government of India (UNFPA, *Saving mother's lives: the challenge continues*).This target aims to bring down the maternal mortality rate by three-quarters by 2015 (Bakshi, 2006).

As noted earlier, substantial evidence is available to guide care practices in the area of episiotomy, labor induction, labor pain management, childbirth support, birthing position, fundal pressure, and communication of information and instructions during labor and delivery. The following is a brief literature review of each of these intrapartum maternity care practices.

Intrapartum Care Practices

In developing countries pregnancy and childbirth complications account for 18% morbidity among females and about 80% of maternal mortality (Bayer, 2004). The deadly pregnancy and childbirth complications included hemorrhage, infection, unsafe abortion, eclampsia, and obstructed labor (World Health Organization, 2000). Inadequate and/ or inappropriate care of women during labor and delivery may lead to one of these deadly intrapartum complications (Sheiner, Sarid, Levy, Seidman, & Hallak, 2005; Everett, Evans, Hutchinson, Collins, & Morrison, 2005). What follows is a list of common labor and delivery practices which may pose a significant health risk to mothers and their offspring.

Episiotomy

The definition of episiotomy is a procedure where the skin between the vagina and the anus (the perineum) is cut. It is done to "enlarge the vaginal opening so that a baby can be more easily delivered" (Medical Encyclopedia, 2005). It is one of the most

15

common surgical procedures done although there is no evidence to support its benefit during childbirth outcome (Lede, Belizan, & Carroli, 1996). Despite the strong body of evidence for restricting the use of episiotomy, unfortunately it is still the most common surgical procedure performed worldwide.

Over the last 100 years, episiotomy has been routinely used by clinicians and historically recommended to facilitate easy delivery of the fetus and to prevent perineal laceration. The rationale for using this procedure was entirely observational, theoretical, and experiential (Graham, 2005). According to Graham (2005), episiotomies were once routinely performed by the doctors in developed countries because they believed it helped to prevent perineal laceration during childbirth. But, as the evidence began to show no benefit of routine episiotomy on maternal outcomes during childbirth, its rate started falling sharply, especially in English speaking countries (Graham, 2005).However, it is still performed often in developing countries (Graham, 2005). Williams, Florey, Mires, & Ogston (1998), in their study found that the rates of episiotomy were significantly higher in women from Indian-subcontinents as compared to white women. This suggests that there is a wide variation in the practice of episiotomy between developing and developed countries (Renfrew, Hannah, Albers, & Floyd, 1998). This persistent wide variation in episiotomy rate signifies that routine use of episiotomy is strongly compelled by local professional norms, experiences during training, and individual preferences rather than variation in the needs of women during childbirth (Hartman et al., 2005). Lack of knowledge and outdated practice habits of care providers' may result in significant use of routine, but ineffective, possibly harmful, use of episiotomies (Wick, et al., 2005).

Lede, et al. (1996) reported that the major justification provided by the professionals for routine use of episiotomy is that it prevents severe perineal lacerations that could contribute to incontinence. It had been anticipated by the care providers that episiotomy would heal more quickly and with fewer complications than a spontaneous tear and women will be less likely to have impaired sexual function later on (Hartman et al., 2005). On the contrary, it was found by Lede, et al. (1996) that the routine use of

16

episiotomy involves a greater need of surgical perineal repair, more maternal discomfort, and poor sexual function. According to Hartman et al. (2005), there is fair to good amount of evidence from a number of clinical trials suggesting that immediate maternal outcomes of routine episiotomy, including severity of perineal laceration, pain and pain medication use are not better than those with restrictive use of episiotomy.

It should be noted that Haadam (1998) found that episiotomy is protective against anterior perineal tears. However, there is no evidence to support the belief that episiotomy protects against anal sphincter tears, pelvic muscle damage or urinary incontinence. Rather women who were subjected to episiotomy were found to have more blood loss, disrupted wound healing, and increased pain during the early puerperium (Haadam, 1998). Women tend to have increased length of hospital stay if they had episiotomy (Hueston, 1996). The infection rate was also found to be higher in women with episiotomies as compared to women who had spontaneous laceration (Larsson, Christensen, Bergman, & Wallstersson, 1991).

The case for restricting the use of episiotomy is conclusive (Renfrew, et al., 1998). Results from randomized controlled trials on restricting the use of episiotomy have shown a 9% reduction in severe perineal tears (Lede, et al., 1996; Low, Seng, Murtland, and Oakley, 2000; AHRQ, 2005; Goldberg & Fagan, 2000-2006). Restricting the use of episiotomy may reduce maternal morbidity due to infection, reduce length of hospital stay, decreased cost of delivery, decrease psychological distress, promote early initiation of breast feeding, decrease posterior perineal trauma, less suturing, and fewer healing complications (Carroli & Belizan, 2000; Qian, et al., 2006).

Labor Induction

Induction of labor is the "artificial initiation of labor before its spontaneous onset for the purpose of delivery of the feto-placental unit" (Crane, 2001, p. 1). The rate of labor induction is high in developed countries. Baxley (2003) reported that the prevalence of labor induction in the United States has nearly doubled over the past decade. Studies

17

have shown that in developing countries the practice of labor induction is seemingly rising (Crane, 2001).

Labor induction is a common obstetric intervention, which should be done only with a specific clinical indication such as post-dated pregnancy, premature rupture of membranes, suspected fetal compromise, and maternal medical problems (British Columbia Reproductive Care, 1998; Summers, 1997). However, it may also be practiced for other reasons such as women's request or clinician's convenience (Howarth & Botha, 2001). It was found in a study conducted in Northern Belgium comparing the outcomes of labor induction in 15,000 healthy and uncomplicated primigravida mothers, that half of the women who requested labor induction used significantly more pain medications, had more cesarean sections due to both fetal distress and stalled labor, and more forceps and vacuum deliveries (Cammu, Martens, Ruyssinck, & Ammy, 2002). Artificially induced labor does not have the same outcomes as spontaneous labor. Mothers whose labors have been induced generally complain of severe pain and may increase the need for epidural analgesia (Cammu, et al., 2002).

Using medications to induce labor for non-medical reasons has attracted both care providers and women for years and the non-medical reasons for elective labor induction includes the mutual convenience of both women and their care providers (Baxley, 2003).

Various studies have reviewed the potential risks for elective induction of labor such as iatrogenic prematurity, uterine hyperstimulation, shoulder dystocia, postpartum hemorrhage, and non-reassuring fetal heart rate, significant increased risk of cesarean delivery in nulliparous women, and increase in-hospital predelivery time and cost (Baxley, 2003; Gail, 2001; Berka, Socol, & Dooley, 1999; Maslow & Sweeney, 2000; Cammu, et al., 2002).

In summary induction of labor still introduces considerable risk compared with natural onset of labor, and many, if not most, inductions are done for reasons that are not supported by sound medical research (Coalition for Improving Maternity Services, 2003).

18

Therefore, based on the evidence available regarding harmful effects of labor induction, WHO (1999) has recommended that labor should not be induced for convenience. Rather, it should be reserved for specific medical induction and no geographic region should have rates of induced labor over 10%. The indication for labor induction should be discussed with women along with the benefits and potential risks and should be considered when it is felt that the benefits of vaginal delivery outweigh the potential maternal and fetal risks of induction (Crane, 2001).

Birthing Position

Maternal position for the second stage of labor has been subject to ritual for many years (Tillett, 2005). There are various birthing positions which are used during the second stage of labor to deliver the baby (Gupta, Hofmeyr, & Smyth, 2004). The position assumed by women during childbirth is highly influenced by several complex factors. For example, practices such as perineal support and instrumental assistance of the birth during spontaneous delivery have restricted options for positions assumed by women (Gupta, et al., 2004).

It is interesting to point out that throughout pregnancy women are told by their care providers not to sleep on their back due to compromised blood flow to the fetus. In contrast, in many countries women are made to lie down on their back during labor and delivery (Johnson, Newburn, & Macfarlane, 2002).The one common reason given by the care providers for encouraging women to be in supine position is that it is easier for them to monitor fetal heart patterns (Gupta, et al., 2004). However, earlier it was found that non-supine position such as side-lying provides prophylaxis against fetal aortocaval compression, thereby helping to improve fetal heart rate (Preston, Crosby, Kotarba, Dudas, & Elliot, 1993).

Previously Gupta & Nikodem (2003), in their systemic review, examined the effects of women's position on the second stage of labor. They found that the use of any non-supine or upright position, as compared to supine or lithotomy position was associated with reduced duration of second stage of labor, reduction in episiotomies, reduced reporting of severe pain, and fewer abnormal fetal heart rate patterns. However, they also found that non-supine or upright position may lead to postpartum hemorrhage due to the likelihood of second degree tear or blood loss greater than 500 ml. The chance of blood loss in the supine position is low but the difference was only significant for multigravidas (Gupta & Nikodem, 2003).

The upright positions such as standing, kneeling, or squatting helps the baby move down while providing the advantage of gravity and widens the diameter of pelvis thereby creating more room for the baby to come out (Johnson, Johnson, & Gupta, 1991; Keene, DiFranco, & Amis, 2005). The side-lying and semi-sitting positions are considered as restful and useful for women who are exhausted and may help to slow down a precipitated labor (Keene, et al., 2005). In light of the available evidence, WHO (1999), recommends women adopt any position they like, while preferably avoiding long periods lying supine, and they should be encourage to experiment with what feels most comfortable and should be supported in their choice.

Continuous Support during Labor

Continuous support during childbirth is one of the important ways to provide a positive childbirth experience for women. Historically and cross-culturally, women have been attended and supported by other women during the childbirth process, especially labor (Hodnett, Gates, Hofmeyr, & Sakala, 2003). However, in recent decades in hospitals worldwide, as childbirth moved out of the home and into the hospital, continuous support during labor has become the exception rather than the routine part of birthing process (Hodnett, et al., 2003). Concerns about the consequence of medicalizing natural childbirth and overlooking women's birth experiences have led to calls for a return to continuous support by women during labor (Hodnett, et al., 2003). However, at present the importance of providing continuous support either from family or caregivers to women during labor is significantly neglected in developing countries like India.

Labor has always been a painful and fearful experience for women. Campero et al., (1998) found that with the continuous presence of a support person. It was easy for women to manage pain and bear down effectively, as the support person acted as a distractor and helped women to manage the pain effectively. Researchers have found that a constant human presence decreases the anxiety, pain, and fear which women generally experience during labor (Hunter, 2002).

The elements of labor support reported for women as helpful and effective for them are emotional support (continuous presence, reassurance, encouragement, and praise); physical support (comfort measures aimed at decreasing hunger, thirst, and pain); information on their labor progress and advice on coping mechanisms; and advocacy (respecting women's decision and helping them to communicate to other healthcare team members) (Hodnett, 1996). These are the elements that are recommended in the literature to be included in the care of a laboring woman as they contribute to decreasing anxiety, pain, and fear, resulting in shorter second stage of labor and presumably better birth experience for women (Hunter, 2002).

In recent years studies have shown that continuous support during labor has a number of benefits with no risks involved. The Cochrane Systematic review of 14 randomized controlled trials of continuous support during childbirth found that women who received continuous intrapartum support had less use of analgesics and anesthetics, less instrumental deliveries, fewer low Apgar scores in their newborns, fewer problems with the coping mechanism during labor, and more satisfaction from their childbirth experience (Hodnett, et al., 2003). Other than these benefits, caregiver support also increased the likelihood of 4-6 weeks of breastfeeding after delivery and better results were reported with post-partum anxiety and self-esteem in women with support (Hodnett, 2002). Kennel, Klaus, Mcgrath, Robertson, & Hinkley (1991), conducted a randomized controlled trial more than a decade ago looking at the outcomes of emotional support during labor in 412 nulliparous women. They found that providing touch, encouragement, information and explanation of procedures to women significantly reduced the rate of cesarean section and forceps delivery. In addition they found decreased use of oxytocin, shorter second stage of labor, and decreased chances of acquiring puerperal sepsis in women provided with social support at the time of labor. Based on their findings, they concluded that continuous support to women was not only emotionally and physically beneficial to them, but it also proved to be cost effective for the hospital.

Therefore, it is imperative to understand and provide who laboring women perceive as most effective support to protect them from the potentially harmful effects of stress during childbirth. Support will only be beneficial when the women sees the support person as valuable, desirable, and useful (Ip, 2000). Because of the benefits of childbirth support, WHO (2003) encourages the constant support from the chosen birth companion by the woman. This person should provide physical and psychological comfort throughout the childbirth process, including help to relax and move around, aid in toileting when needed, encouragement to drink fluids and eat as she wishes, as well as support using local practices.

Fundal Pressure

Fundal pressure is described as an "external force applied at the uppermost portion of the uterus in a caudal direction typically with the intent of shortening the duration of the second stage of labor" (Buhimschi, Buhimischi, Malino, Kopelman, & Weiner, 2002, p. 520). It is considered as one of the most controversial maneuvers that are used in the second stage of labor (Merhi and Awonuga, 2005). In many countries the care givers commonly practice fundal pressure during the second stage of labor in order to help to expedite the delivery process and shorten the second stage of labor (WHO, 1999). There is very limited data on the subject of its safety and efficacy (Merhi & Awonuga, 2005).

In 1990, Kline-Kaye & Miller found that 84% of the care- givers reported using fundal pressure during the second stage of labor. The reasons given for this intervention include fetal distress, maternal exhaustion, risk of cesarean delivery, and effects of

22

regional anesthesia. Historically, description of the use of fundal pressure for cesarean section, shoulder dystocia, and during third stage management can be found in the literature but very limited information is available for practicing fundal pressure in second stage of labor for other indications (Oxorn, 1986).

The risks associated with the use of fundal pressure have been described by Cosner (1996). These risks included a longer duration of second stage of labor and increased third- and fourth degree perineal tear in women who had fundal pressure as compared to those with spontaneous delivery. The possible association of other maternal complications, including abdominal bruising, uterine inversion, hypotension, respiratory distress, liver rupture, fractured ribs, and pain are of significant concern. Fetal risks include abnormal fetal heart rate, neurological, and orthopedic disorders, fetal hypoxemia, and intracranial hemorrhage (Simpson and Knox, 2001). One of the rarest but more serious complications that could happen due to fundal pressure is uterine rupture (Kline-Kaye & Miller, 1990). Kline-Kaye & Miller reported that uterine ruptures occurred in scarred uterus as compared to unscarred uterus. In a study of 63 women with scarred uterus from previous cesarean section, there was a reported uterine rupture in half of the women who received fundal pressure during delivery. Thus, fundal pressure along with forceps and oxytocin use was considered an iatrogenic factor for uterine rupture (Vangeenderhuysen & Souidi, 2002).

Despite the dogma "never fundal pressure," a high percentage of medical institutions use it (Merhi & Awonuga, 2005). But the prevalence of the use of fundal pressure is probably underreported as it was noted that a majority of care givers did not document this procedure. Perhaps as a reflection of the controversial nature of fundal pressure, obstetricians may not document their performance of this procedure and the fear of litigation may contribute to the failure of physicians as well as nurses to document this procedure (Merhi & Awonuga, 2005). It is important for the care providers to judiciously examine the importance of fundal pressure during second stage of labor and to evaluate its effectiveness based on the women's condition.

Overall there is little evidence support the use of fundal pressure during second stage of labor. Therefore, WHO (1999) describes fundal pressure during second stage of labor as a practice which has insufficient evidence to support a clear recommendation and therefore it should be used with caution while further research clarifies the issue.

Labor Pain Management

World wide, pain management during the childbirth process is one of the major concerns for women and their care providers. Women experience a wide range of pain in labor and exhibit an equally wide range of responses towards it (World Health Organization, 2005). A number of pharmacological and non-pharmacological methods are available today to manage pain during labor. However, little attention has been paid towards considering its efficacy and safety as well as access to women's choice of pain relief methods.

Pharmacological methods commonly employed during labor are parenteral opioids and epidurals. Parenteral opioids have been in use for decades, but there remains conflicting information regarding their safety and efficacy when used as labor analgesia (Leeman, Fontaine, King, Klien, & Ratcliffe, 2003). In developed countries, epidural analgesia is frequently used during labor as compared to developing countries. Patients' requests and caregivers' perceptions in developed countries towards the use of analgesia have resulted in a substantial increase in the use of epidural analgesia during childbirth over the past two decades (Robert, Vincent, & Chestnut, 1998). Epidural anesthetics theoretically could reduce 100 percent of labor pain if used in large doses and high concentrations (Robert, et al. 1998). However, the use of epidurals during labor presents significant drawbacks. First, it may take longer for the baby to rotate and descend. The use of epidural analgesia may decrease the sense of pain which can interfere with the natural release of oxytocin, which can cause a drop in women's blood pressure and may affect the fetal heart rate. The regional numbness may affect the women's bladder and lead to urinary retention. Most importantly, an epidural may lead to

24

a higher rate of instrumental delivery and longer labor especially with primigravida mothers (Lothian, Amis, & Crenshaw, 2005). Similar findings were reported in the systematic review of 21 randomized control trials on "epidurals and non-epidurals in labor". (Anim, Smyth, & Howell, 2005). Although pain relief with epidural analgesia is reported to be effective, it hampers other desired goals such as walking during the first stage of labor and pushing effectively during second stage (Leeman, et al., 2003). As an alternative to epidural analgesia, parenteral opioid analgesics do relieve labor pain for one to two hours. However, with the use of parenteral opioid analgesia there is a subsequent increase in the use of epidural analgesia as well as side-effects including nausea and vomiting, increased cesarean deliveries, instrumental assisted vaginal deliveries, and maternal exhaustion during second stage of labor (Bricker & Lavender, 2002).

Several randomized controlled trials have compared parenteral opioids with epidural analgesia. Bricker & Lavender (2002), found that lower rates of oxytocin use, shorter second stage labor, less cases of fetal malpositions, and decreased number of instrumental deliveries were reported in women who received parenteral opioids during labor. However, the level of pain relief and maternal satisfaction was reported to be high in women with epidural analgesia as compared to parenteral opioids (Sharma et al., 1997).

Non-pharmacological methods of labor pain relief include a wide variety of techniques such as patterned breathing, mental imaging, massage or therapeutic touch, warm baths and showers, music, and local application of heat and cold (Albers, 1998). Albers found in the observational study that women who received epidurals and intrathecal narcotics had a significantly lower rate of spontaneous delivery as compared to those who received non-pharmacological measures of pain relief. Non-pharmacological labor pain relief methods have been traditionally used throughout history. Despite the fact that these methods reduce pain, provide comfort, and reduce the chances of other morbid maternal and neonatal outcomes, they have received limited

25

attention in both developed and developing countries. The challenges of providing pain relief for women in labor and birth are complex and delivering regional anesthesia to control the pain may not be the only answer. Women should be aware of all the options available to them when it comes to managing pain during labor (WHO, 2005).

Communication of Information and Instructions

Information and instructions provided to women during the childbirth process, especially during the intrapartum phase, may be helpful to women in labor. Women want to be informed of their progress of labor and baby's condition (Bowers, 2002). To ensure support and communication during childbirth, it is necessary that care providers explain all procedures, seek permission, and discuss findings with women. As well, a supportive and encouraging atmosphere for birth is necessary. Coaching provided to women during childbirth has both physiological and psychological benefits for women. A study was conducted which compared obstetrical outcomes associated with coached versus uncoached pushing during second stage of labor (Bloom, Casey, Schatter, McIntire, & Leveno, 2006). Researches found that out of 320 nulliparous women 163 women who received instructions and information on pushing and breathing technique did not ask for epidural analgesia or required oxytocin as well as had reduce second stage of labor as compared to uncoached mothers. Respecting women's wishes as well as maintaining privacy and confidentiality is considered foundational to high quality intrapartum care (Damanhoury, Azzam, & Ibrahim, 2003).

The importance of a supportive labor companion and timely, accurate information is highly valued in developed countries. However, in developing countries the usual standard is more likely authoritative care and minimal information sharing with women about their progress of labor. A study conducted in Mexico examined the experiences of mothers who received psychosocial support from a doula and compared them with the experiences of those women who gave birth following normal hospital routine (Campero et al., 1998). Sixteen in-depth interviews were held with women in the immediate post partum period. It was found that women who did not receive any support reported that they perceived the information provided to them by the caregivers authoritative and discouraging of their abilities to clarify their concerns or ask questions regarding their labor progress. These researchers found that a lack of or inconsistent information makes the childbirth experience worse for women as fear and unreflected knowledge seemed to block their acquisition of new knowledge (Hallgren, Kihlgren, Norberg, & Forslin, 1995). When opinions and choices are not provided to women during childbirth, women assume that whatever procedure is done to them are expected norms and routinely practiced.

Laboring women want to be considered as individuals, expect to have a trusting relationship with their care providers, and want to be supported and guided through their own choices of childbirth (Berg, Laundgren, Hermansson, & Wahlberg, 1996). Reflecting the importance of communicating information and providing instructions to women during childbirth, WHO (1999) recommended that care providers should give information and explanations as much as women request and need.

Difference in Care Providers' Opinions and Practices

A number of studies have been done looking into the difference in maternity care provided by different types of clinicians such as physicians, midwives, nurse-midwives, and nurses practices in developed countries such as the United States, but no such studies were found that examined these differences in India. Overall, in the developed world, there seems to be a difference between the medical model that considers labor as a medical process with high potential for complications and the midwifery model that perceives labor as a normal process and as much possible should be treated normally with no medical interventions (Steer, 1999). The "midwifery model" of care is supported by various studies where it has been found that care provided by nurse-midwives as compared to physicians, has excellent outcomes with lower rates of interventional deliveries, labor induction, and cesarean section (Knedle-Murray, Oakley, Wheeler, & Peterson, 1993; Public Citizen's Health Research Group, 1995). These findings have

27

been supported by more recent work by Reime, et al. in 2004. These researchers compared the self-reported practices, attitudes and beliefs about issues in childbirth including routine electronic fetal monitoring, labor induction, epidural analgesia, episiotomy, doulas, and vaginal birth after cesarean section. Based on their findings, they concluded that obstetricians favored technology and interventions during normal childbirth as compared to midwives. However, it was difficult for the researchers to generalize the findings because obstetricians and midwives follow a different approach towards normal childbirth care.

In summary, there are care practices employed during childbirth which have been found to be harmful for both mothers and babies. These include episiotomy, use of oxytocics for labor augmentation, parenteral narcotics, giving birth in lithotomy position, inadequate and inappropriate communication of information to mothers regarding the care, and not allowing women to have continuous support or companion during labor and delivery. These customary practices are not congruent with the recommendations of WHO in spite of universal access to the recommendations put forth by WHO. Even after knowing the facts and effectiveness of evidence-based childbirth care, it is often difficult for the care providers to overcome their beliefs and rituals. However, to improve the maternal health outcomes, maternity care providers must begin to base their practice on evidence, not ritual. This is the way to save women's lives.

CHAPTER III

METHODOLOGY

This chapter describes the design and methods used for this research study, including the sampling technique employed, a description of the instrument used, the data collection procedure, and the protection of human subjects. The goal of this study was to describe the opinions and current care practice of maternity care providers. Therefore, a survey research format was chosen and constructed using both closed and open ended questions.

The purpose of this study was to survey maternity care providers (nurse-midwives and doctors) as to their opinions and self-report of current intrapartum care practices and to compare these self reported practices with the WHO recommendations. The research questions were as follows:

1. What are the intrapartum care practices as reported by the respondents? including episiotomy, labor induction, childbirth support, labor pain management, fundal pressure, birthing position, and communication of information and instructions to women during intrapartum phase.

2. How do these reported intrapartum care practices compare with the WHO practice guidelines?

3. What are the differences in the intrapartum care practices between doctors and nurse-midwives?

4. What are the differences in the intrapartum care practices between government and non-government hospitals?

Sample

A non-probability, convenience sample was used for this study. Only nurse-midwives and obstetricians who were currently practicing childbirth care were included in the study. A total of 250 maternity care providers were given surveys and 188 were returned to the researcher. The care providers worked in Government and Non-Government hospitals of New Delhi and Rajasthan.

Instruments

A semi-structured survey questionnaire was developed to reflect opinions and current care practices of maternity care providers, with 34 items in the form of fixed-choice and open ended questions. The survey questions concerning the key points of intrapartum care management were drawn from the researcher's personal observations and from studying the relevant literature. As well, the survey developed by Wick, et al. was also adapted for this study. Permission to use their instrument was granted by the researcher. The questionnaire was reviewed by one content expert and revised for ease of use and understanding.

The survey asks demographic and practice related questions addressing intrapartum care management issues. Demographic information requested for this study included their professional category, work experience, and type of hospital they belong. Categories of questions reflecting intrapartum management issues address the self-reported practices and personal preferences for the routine practices of episiotomy, labor induction, labor pain management, support during labor and delivery, delivery position, communication of information and instructions during labor and delivery, and fundal pressure. The complete questionnaire is found in Appendix A.

Procedure

A questionnaire was developed to explore the opinions and current care practice of maternity care providers during intrapartum period of childbirth process. A survey method was used to collect data from the participants. The developed questionnaire was personally handed out to the participants during December 2005 and January 2006. Each questionnaire was included with a permission letter and a cover letter stating the researcher's background, purpose, confidentiality, and anonymity assurance for the participants for the study (See Appendix B). The survey was estimated to take 15-30 minutes to complete.

Upon obtaining permission from selected hospitals, participants were personally approached and this researcher requested their participation in the survey. A total 250 questionnaires were distributed to the participants. Follow up reminders were given verbally to all participants to achieve maximum responses. The study received a 75.2% (188/250) response rate. Weekly follow-ups were done by the researcher to collect data. Data collection took place from 12/12/05 to 01/20/06. Collected data were brought back from India to University of New Hampshire by the researcher.

Human Subjects

The research proposal for the study was approved by the UNH Institutional Review Board (IRB). The consent form was prepared and matched with the University of New Hampshire standards. Confidentiality of the participants' information was assured at all phases of the research. There were no known risks to participants in the study. There were no financial benefits provided to the participants for participating in the study. However, the study might help the participants to reflect on their practice, to expand the body of knowledge related to the significance of evidence-based practice and promote adherence to set standards of practice provided by WHO. Participants who requested an abstract of this study were assured by researcher that they will receive a copy of abstract and, if interested, can get more details of findings, after completion of the study

CHAPTER IV.

DATA ANALYSIS

The findings of this survey are presented in this section. The purpose of this study was to address the following research questions:

1. What are the intrapartum care practices as reported by the respondents? including episiotomy, labor induction, childbirth support, labor pain management, fundal pressure, birthing position, and communication of information and instructions to women during intrapartum phase.

2. How do these reported intrapartum care practices compare with the WHO practice guidelines?

3. What are the differences in the intrapartum care practices between doctors and nurse-midwives?

4. What are the differences in the intrapartum care practices between government and non-government hospitals?

The obtained data from the participants was first recorded into EXCEL sheet as a spreadsheet. Data from the EXCEL spreadsheet was then entered into Statistical Package for the Social Sciences (SPSS 14), which was used for final data analysis.

Sample Demographics

A total of 188 eligible participants' doctors and nurse-midwives from different government and non-government hospitals of New Delhi and Rajasthan comprised the subjects in this survey-based study. A total of 157 (83.5%) of the participants in the study consisted of nurse-midwives. Most (90.2%) of these nurse-midwives were from government hospitals (Table 1). The doctors who participated in the survey had a wide range of experience, between 1 to 27 years with a mean of 9.7 years. Nurse-midwives reported experience ranged 1 to 20 years with a mean of 3.9 years.

32

Table 1
Demographics

	Count	%	Doctors (n = 31) Count	%	Nurse-midwives (n = 157) Count	%
Participants (N = 188)						
Government	123	65.4	12	9.8	111	90.2
Non-government	53	28.2	16	30.2	37	69.8
X *	12	6.4	3	25	9	30.2

Note: * Non-identified hospitals

When asked "who attends normal birth at their work place"? Half of the
participants reported that both doctors and nurse-midwives equally involved in attending
normal childbirth (Table 2).

Table 2
 Frequency Distribution for Birth Attending Personnel

Group	Count	%
	(N = 187)	
Doctors	62	33
Nurse-midwives	30	16
Both	95	50.5

Participants were asked whether their practice is based on any recommended
policy or protocols (Table 3). It is interesting to note that about equal number of
participants reported that they "don't know" about the policy for their current practice and
they "don't have" any written policy for normal childbirth.

Table 3
Frequency Distribution for Written Clinical Practice Policy

Written policy	Count	%
	(N = 178)	
Yes	82	43.6
No	44	23.4
Don't know	52	27.7

33

Research Q 1: - Reported Intrapartum Care Practices

Participants were asked their opinion whether "episiotomies should be performed for nearly all deliveries, nearly all primigravidas, and anyone who would tear", on a 4 point Likert scale. It was found that the mean score of participants' responses on their opinion towards conducting episiotomy for nearly all deliveries fell for "strongly disagree" whereas the responses for conducting episiotomy to all primigravidas' and anyone who would tear were laying between "strongly agree" and "agree" on Likert scale. The mean scores are reported in Table 4.

Table 4
Frequency Distribution for Opinion towards Episiotomy

Variable	Strongly agree %	Agree %	Strongly disagree %	Disagree %	$\overline{X}$	SD
Nearly all deliveries (n = 165)	9	5.9	36.7	36.2	3.14	.936
All primigravidas (n = 180)	43.6	46.8	4.3	1.1	1.61	.629
Anyone who would tear (n = 172)	53.7	31.4	4.8	1.6	1.50	.680

When participants were asked "how often do they perform episiotomy on primigravida and multigravida mothers"? The findings showed that more than half of the respondents reported they always perform episiotomy for primigravida mothers (Table 5).

Table 5
Frequency Distribution for Episiotomy Practice

Groups	Always %	Frequently %	Sometimes %	Rarely %	Never %	$\overline{X}$	SD
Primigravida (n = 188)	74.5	24.5	___	___	1.1	1.29	.578
Multigravida (n=166)	1.6	12.8	51.6	19.7	2.7	3.10	.744

It was also found that care providers generally do not consider mother's preference while deciding episiotomy use (Table 6).

Table 6
Frequency Distribution for Considering Womens' Preference for Episiotomy

Groups	Count	%
	(N=182)	
Yes	31	16.5
No	130	69.1
Unable to answer	21	11.2

Next, participants were asked whether episiotomy or perineal laceration caused more discomfort and vulval-hematoma formation. Interestingly, more than half of the participants reported that perineal laceration causes more discomfort and vulval-hematoma formation as compared to episiotomy (Table 7).

Table 7
Frequency Distribution for Discomfort and Vulval-hematoma Formation

Variable	Discomfort (n = 186)		Vulval hematoma (n = 185)	
	Count	%	Count	%
Episiotomy	22	11.7	39	20.7
Perineal laceration	126	67	123	65.4
Both equally	38	20.2	23	12.2

Nearly half of the participants (Table 8) reported that they use drugs for labor pain relief. Only 15% of 84 subjects mentioned using epidural for pain relief during labor. More than half of the participants reported that they use non-pharmacological methods for relieving labor pain (Table 8).

Table 8
Frequency Distribution for Labor Pain Relief Methods

	Pharmacological (n = 185)		Non-pharmacological (n = 159)	
	Count	%	Count	%
Yes	93	49.5	119	63.3
No	92	48.9	40	21.3

The mean percentage for primigravida and multigravida mothers receiving pharmacological and non-pharmacological pain relief measures are reported in Table 9.

Table 9
Mean Percentage for women receiving Pain Relief Measures

Groups	Pharmacological		Non-pharmacological	
	X	SD	X	SD
Primigravida	56.8	30.8	61.7	30.5
	(n = 72)		(n = 50)	
Multigravida	38.2	26.9	59.7	34.7
	(n = 69)		(n = 47)	

In response to the question "In your institution, how often does the mother deliver in the following position: lithotomy, semi-sitting, lateral, upright, and squatting"? Nearly all participants reported that they always use the lithotomy position with women during the delivery process (Table 10). Birthing position such as upright, squatting, semi-sitting, and lateral were not often used by the care providers in their care practice.

Table 10
Frequency Distribution for Birthing Position

Variables	Always %	Frequently %	Sometimes %	Rarely %	Never %	X̄	SD
Lithotomy (n =183)	91	4.3	2.1	___	___	1.1	.3
Semi-sitting (n = 137)	2.7	5.3	11.7	8	45.2	4.2	1.2
Lateral (n = 124)	___	3.7	3.2	3.7	55.3	4.7	.8
Upright (n = 125)	___	___	.5	7.4	58.5	4.9	.3
Squatting (n = 130)	1.1	___	2.1	4.3	61.7	4.8	.6

Next, the participants were asked to report whether they induce labor routinely or not? Interestingly, participants reported inducing labor as a routine procedure (Table 11). It was also found that drugs alone were more often used for labor induction as compared to AROM alone (Artificial Rupture of Membranes) or both AROM & drugs in combination (Table 11).

Table 11
Frequency Distribution for Labor Induction

Variables	Count	%
Routine labor induction (n = 184)		
Yes	70	37.2
No	114	60.6
Method (n = 107)		
Drugs	41	21.8
AROM	33	17.6
Both	33	17.6

Based on the participants' practice experience, mean percentage of receiving drugs for labor induction was reported higher in low risk primigravida mothers as compared to multigravida mothers (Table 12).

37

Table 12
Mean Percentage of Low Risk Women Receiving Labor Induction

Groups	Drugs		ARM	
	X	SD	X	SD
Primigravida	55.5	22.3	51.2	25
	(n = 74)		(n = 60)	
Multigravida	39.3	23.7	51.8	25.7
	(n = 70)		(n = 64)	

Even though the application of fundal pressure carries significant risk and is often a hidden clinical intervention, more than a quarter of the respondents reported applying fundal pressure "sometimes" on primigravida mothers (Table13).

Table 13
Frequency Distribution for Practicing Fundal Pressure

Groups	Always %	Frequently %	Sometimes %	Rarely %	Never %	X	SD
Primigravida (n = 181)	3.2	18.1	38.8	29.3	6.9	3.2	.9
Multigravida (n = 173)	3.7	3.7	19.7	52.1	12.8	3.7	.9

When asked whether they provide information during labor and delivery on a routine basis, a majority responded that they "always" provide information to mothers during the intrapartum phase (Table 14).

Table 14
Frequency Distribution for Routine Information

Variable	Always %	Frequently %	Sometimes %	Rarely %	Never %	X
Routine information (N = 175)	69.1	20.2	3.2	.5	____	1.3

However supportive the respondents may be in providing information, the majority of the care providers do not allow mothers to have a support person of her choice during the labor and delivery process (Table 15).

Table 15
Frequency distribution for support person

Support person (N = 174)	Count	%
Yes	34	18.1
No	140	74.5

Research Q 2:- Comparison of Findings with WHO Guidelines on

Intrapartum Care Practices

The findings of reported intrapartum care practices were compared with WHO recommendations and reported in Table 16.

Table 16
Comparison of study findings with WHO guidelines

Practices	WHO Guidelines	Study Findings
Episiotomy	The systematic use of episiotomy is not justified. The protection of the perineum through other methods should be evaluated and adopted.	Episiotomy was found to be practiced by care-providers for primigravida mothers. (Table 5)
Labor induction	Birth should not be induced for convenience. No geographic region should have rates of induced labor more than 10%. Induction should match the criteria of its indication.	Labor induction was found to be commonly employed by the care providers for primigravida mothers. (Table 12)
Birthing position	Pregnant women should not be put in lithotomy position during labor and delivery. They should be encouraged to freely decide which position they would like to be comfortable in delivery process.	Nearly every participant reported that they always put mother in lithotomy position while conducting deliveries. (Table 10)
Fundal pressure	WHO describes fundal pressure during second stage of labor as a practice which has insufficient evidence to support a clear recommendation and therefore it should be used with caution while further research clarifies the issue.	Application of fundal pressure was found to be higher in primigravidas' as compared to multigravida mothers. (Table 13)
Childbirth support	WHO encourages the constant support from the chosen birth companion by the women who should provide physical and psychological comfort through out the childbirth process such as help her to relax and moving around, take her to toilet when needed, encourage her to drink fluids and eat as she wishes, give support using local practices, and do other supportive actions.	In practice, choice to have continuous support was not given to mothers during labor and delivery. (Table 15)
Labor pain management	During delivery, the routine administration of analgesic or anesthetic drugs, that are not specifically required to correct or prevent a complication in delivery, should be avoided.	Findings reported that care providers frequently use pharmacological methods to manage labor pain during childbirth process. (Table 8)
Routine Information	Women should receive as much information as they desire.	Majority of the participants reported providing information to women during labor and delivery. (Table 14)

Research Q 3:- Difference in the Intrapartum Care Practices between Doctors and

Nurse-Midwives

To find out the differences in care practices of between doctors and nurse-midwives, data were grouped by profession. Analysis of variance (ANOVA) was performed to measure the significant differences in mean scores between the groups.

There was no significant difference found between doctors and nurse-midwives in their opinion towards conducting episiotomy (Table 17). Both the groups agreed that episiotomy should be performed for nearly all primigravidas and to those who would tear.

Table: 17
Mean Opinions toward Episiotomy Practice in Professional Group

| Variable | Doctors | | Nurse-midwives | | F ratio | p |
	Mean	SD	Mean	SD		
Episiotomy to all deliveries	3.1	.7	3.1	.9	.007	.932
	(n = 26)		(n= 139)			
Episiotomy to all primigravida	1.5	.5	1.6	.6	.769	.382
	(n = 29)		(n = 151)			
Episiotomy who would tear	1.5	.6	1.5	.7	.092	.762
	(n = 28)		(n = 144)			

Significant differences in mean scores were found in the practice of applying fundal pressure and birthing position (semi-sitting) between doctors and nurse-midwives (Table 18). Doctors reported practicing semi-sitting position "sometimes" whereas nurse-midwives "rarely" use this position for delivering baby. The findings suggest that both groups had strong practice behavior for providing lithotomy position to women during childbirth.

No significant difference was found in the practice of episiotomy between nurse-midwives and doctors (Table 18). Both the groups reported doing "frequent" episiotomy for primigravida and "sometimes" for multigravida mothers.

41

Table: 18
Mean Practice of Episiotomy, Fundal Pressure, and Birthing Position in Professional Group

Variable	Doctors Mean	SD	Nurse-midwives Mean	SD	F ratio	p
Episiotomy						
Primigravida	1.2 (n = 31)	.4	1.3 (n = 157)	.6	.418	.519
Multigravida	2.9 (n = 31)	.6	3.1 (n = 135)	.7	1.252	.265
Fundal pressure						
Primigravida	2.4 (n = 30)	.8	3.3 (n = 151)	.9	29.880	.000
Multigravida	3.2 (n = 29)	.9	3.8 (n = 144)	.8	12.240	.001
Birthing position						
Lithotomy	1.2 (n = 29)	.5	1.1 (n = 154)	.3	4.026	.046
Sem-sitting	3.5 (n = 20)	1.2	4.3 (n = 117)	1.1	8.981	.003
Lateral	4.9 (n = 15)	.2	4.6 (n = 109)	.8	1.705	.194
Upright	5.0 (n = 15)	.0	4.8 (n = 110)	.4	2.192	.141
Squatting	4.9 (n = 15)	.3	4.8 (n = 115)	.6	.111	.740

Again, a significant difference was found between nurse-midwives and doctors in their opinion about whether episiotomy causes more formation of vulval-hematoma as compared to perineal laceration (Table 19).

Table: 19
Mean Perception for Cause of Discomfort and Vulval-hematoma in Professional Group

Variable	Doctors Mean	SD	Nurse-midwives Mean	SD	F ratio	p
Discomfort	2.2 (n = 30)	.5	2.0 (n = 156)	.5	2.469	.118
Vulval-hematoma	1.7 (n = 30)	.5	1.9 (n = 155)	.5	5.064	.026

42

Research Q 4:- Difference in the Intrapartum Care Practices of

Professionals in Government and Non-Government Hospitals

To find the difference in the care practices of professionals based on the type of hospital, data were grouped by "hospitals". ANOVA was performed to find if there was significant difference between the two groups.

The study found significant differences between government and non-government care providers' opinion towards episiotomy use to all deliveries and all primigravidas (Table 20).

Table: 20
Mean Preference of Episiotomy Practice in Hospital Group

Variable	Government Mean SD		Non-government Mean SD		F ratio	p
Episiotomy to all deliveries	3.4 (n = 107)	.6	2.4 (n = 47)	1.0	44.595	.000
Episiotomy to all primigravida	1.6 (n = 120)	.5	1.3 (n = 49)	.6	9.456	.002
Episiotomy who would tear	1.4 (n = 114)	.5	1.5 (n = 48)	.7	1.404	.238

Care providers from government and non-government hospitals had significant differences in their practices of performing fundal pressure in multigravida mothers and use of birth position. No significant mean difference was found for episiotomy practice (Table 21). Care providers from both types of hospitals had similar practice behavior for all birthing positions except for lithotomy, semi-sitting, lateral, and upright position.

43

Table: 21
Mean Practice of Episiotomy, Fundal Pressure, and Birthing Position in
Hospital group

Variable	Government Mean	SD	Non-government Mean	SD	F ratio	p
Episiotomy						
Primigravida	1.2	.4	1.2	.8	.244	.622
	(n =123)		(n =53)			
Multigravida	3.1	.7	3.0	.8	.336	.563
	(n = 110)		(n = 44)			
Fundal pressure						
Primigravida	3.1	.8	3.1	1.0	.018	.892
	(n = 117)		(n = 52)			
Multigravida	3.8	.8	3.4	1.0	4.936	.028
	(n = 112)		(n = 49)			
Birthing position						
Lithotomy	1.0	.3	1.2	.5	5.654	.019
	(n = 119)		(n = 52)			
Semi-sitting	4.5	1.0	3.4	1.2	26.235	.000
	(n = 92)		(n = 37)			
Lateral	4.9	.4	4.1	1.2	25.374	.000
	(n = 87)		(n = 31)			
Upright	4.9	.2	4.7	.5	7.404	.008
	(n = 87)		(n = 32)			
Squatting	4.7	.7	4.8	.4	.645	.424
	(n = 90)		(n = 34)			

44

Responses to Open-ended Questions

The open ended responses were entered in an EXCEL file rather than SPSS software. This part of the data was not analyzed on the basis of professional or hospital groups. Responses were analyzed for similarity and then categorized. When asked to specify on what standards their written policy concerning normal birth are based only 13% (n = 25) of the total 188 participants responded to this question. Interestingly, 8% (n = 2) of the 25 respondents specified that they follow WHO standards and the remainder mentioned having their own hospital policies for managing normal birth.

When asked why they do not consider mothers' preference for conducting an episiotomy, 56% (n = 106) of the subjects responded. Answers to this open ended question included statements about ignorant and illiterate mothers, doctors' decision, for the well-being of the mother and baby, not mentioned in routine policy, not considered as important to explain, no time to explain, and depends on condition of the mother and baby.

For the question "What are the benefits or drawbacks of episiotomy vs. laceration of same depth?" the majority (77%, n = 145) of the participants mentioned that episiotomy has more benefits as compared to a laceration of the same depth. The episiotomy was believed to heal easily, prevent tears, help the delivery of the baby, causes less pain, have less chance of hematoma formation, and easy to suture.

When asked what drugs they may use for pain relief during the first stage of labor, of the total 188 participants only 84 (45%) responded that they may use drugs such as tramadol, buscopan, phenergan, fortwin, and pethidine. Out of 84 participants, only 14 (17%) reported using epidurals for labor pain relief. In contrast, 109 (58%) participants reported employing deep breathing technique, psychological support, and reassurance as common non-pharmacological methods to relieve labor pain in conjunction with pharmacological methods. For pain relief, the common drugs reported by 92% (n = 173) of the participants used for inducing labor were cervigel, syntocin, epidosin, and misoprostal.

One of the interesting findings of this study was in response to the question, "What do you think is the preferred birthing position for the mothers to deliver?" The majority (88%,n = 165) of the participants answered "lithotomy" and the reasons given for preferring this birthing position included that it is easy for the mothers to deliver, comfortable for the mothers, convenient for the care providers, easy to bear down, and easy to examine the perineum during labor and delivery.

When asked to list the information they provide to mothers during first and second stage of labor and delivery, a total of 130 (69%) participants listed common information. During the first stage of labor they reported providing the following information to mothers:

1. Do not push during contractions.
2. Take deep breaths during contractions.
3. Lie down in left lateral position.
4. Drink lots of fluids.

The following information was reported to be provided during second stage of labor:

1. Push during contractions only.
2. Take deep breaths in between contractions.

To ask about providing constant presence and support during labor and delivery, participants were asked two questions. The first question was asked to specify who remains with the mother. A total of 17 (9%) participants responded to this question and mentioned that it is generally decided by the woman. The second question was to find out whether the support person remains with the mother during labor and delivery. Interestingly, only 3% (n = 6) of the respondents reported that they allow non-clinician presence and support during the first stage of labor.

CHAPTER V

DISCUSSION OF THE FINDINGS

The purpose of this study was to address the following research questions:

1. What are the intrapartum care practices as reported by the respondents? including episiotomy, labor induction, childbirth support, labor pain management, fundal pressure, birthing position, and communication of information and instructions to women during intrapartum phase.

2. How do these reported intrapartum care practices compare with the WHO practice guidelines?

3. What are the differences in the intrapartum care practices between doctors and nurse-midwives?

4. What are the differences in the intrapartum care practices between government and non-government hospitals?

Overall, this study of self-reported intrapartum care practices found that Indian nurse-midwives and physicians do not follow the recommendations of WHO (1996). It appears that self-reported care practices do not reflect the application of current best practice standards. These findings are similar to other reports of maternity care in developing countries, which has found that unproven interventions are widely used while safe and effective care practices are often neglected (Khasholian, 2005). Khasholian conducted a study to document evidence-based care for normal labor and delivery in Egypt, Lebanon, the West bank, and Syria. It was found in the study that many practices that should be eliminated from routine care according to the standards of WHO (1996) were frequently used during normal labor and delivery.

This study found that the lithotomy position is preferred by Indian care providers because they believe that it is comfortable, easy for women to bear down and facilitates the delivery of the baby. This contrast with the evidence that demonstrates birthing positions such as being upright, semi-sitting, squatting, and side lying are safer than the

47

lithotomy position for both mother and fetus (Gupta and Nikodem, 2003). The beneficial effects of not being supine during delivery includes lower rates of episiotomies as well as decreased analgesia and oxytocin use during labor (Bodner et al., 2003; Shorten, Donsante, & Shorten, 2002). However, care providers report that they prefer women to deliver in the lithotomy or supine position as they believe that it is convenient for them to monitor the fetal heart rate. This is in direct contrast with the findings that the supine position is more uncomfortable for mothers and associated with more abnormal fetal heart rates (Gupta, Hofmeyr, & Smyth, 2004).

Along with the persistent use of lithotomy position, another interesting finding of this study was the predominant use of episiotomy during childbirth. Episiotomy, in contrast to current best evidence was routinely employed. The mean score for care providers' opinion towards episiotomy fell in the mid-range between "strongly agree" and "agree" for all primigravida mothers and for those who would be at risk for perineal tear. This finding was not unexpected as the incidence of episiotomy is high in India (Noronha, 2004). It is often found that care providers in developing countries continue to apply a policy of "avoid tears-do episiotomies" routinely (Maduma-Butshe, Dayall, & Garner, 1998). The participants of this study described the reasons for conducting episiotomies as it heals easy than a tear, promotes easy delivery, less painful for the mothers, easy to suture, and less chances of the development of a vulval-hematoma. As this study shows, entrenched experience may trump the best evidence (Low, Seng, Murtlant, and Oakley, 2000). Women may experience fewer potential complications when care givers are able to incorporate scientific evidence in their clinical practices (Signorello, 2000).

Of note there were significant differences found between the practices of care providers in government and non-government hospitals. Care givers from government institutions reported doing episiotomies "frequently" whereas care providers from non-government institutions report performing episiotomies "always" for primigravidas.

As for an evidence-based approach for pain management during labor and delivery the frequent use of opioid analgesics for labor pain relief was reported in this

48

survey. Drugs like tramadol, buscopan, phenergan, pethidine, and fortwin were commonly used for pain relief during labor. Again, these findings reflect a lack of uptake into practice of current best evidence. Opioid analgesics such as pethidine have been associated with fetal respiratory distress and shorter duration of breastfeeding (Caton, Corry, Frigoletto, Hopkins, & Mayberry, 2002). The use of opioid analgesics was reported by the study respondents as less likely to be effective when compared with non-pharmacological methods such as hot and cold therapy and frequent position changing for labor pain relief, which is similar to other studies (Declercq, Sakala, Corry, Applebaum, & Risher, 2002).

Self-report of labor induction practices also did not reflect the WHO standards. The mean percentage of labor induction using drugs and ARM was reported as high for low risk primigravida mothers in this study. The common drugs reported by the care givers for inducing labor were cervigel, syntocin, epidosin, and misoprostal. An early study in 1995 found that in developing countries the frequent use of drugs such as oxytocin during the first stage of labor increased the fetal morbidity and mortality rate (Dujardin et al., 1995). Other complications have been identified that are also associated with labor induction. These include significant discomfort to mothers due to uterine hyperstimulation, maternal fever, increased chances of instrumental deliveries, and episiotomy (Simpson & Atterbury, 2003). It appears that the choice of labor induction to low risk mothers may be based on the convenience factor in order to expedite the delivery process. However, it is important for the care providers to weigh the benefits of labor induction against associated potential maternal and fetal complications (American College of Obstetricians and Gynecologists, 1999). As well, ARM is as equally used as drugs by Indian care providers for labor induction. Although ARM does not have significant risk for laboring mothers' health, it is associated with potential risks for the fetus such as prolapsed umbilical cord, intra-amniotic infection, fetal injury, and uncertain fetal outcomes after delivery (Hadi, 2000; Usta, Mercer, & Sibai, 1999; American College of Obstetricians and Gynecologists, 1999).

Next, a significant difference in the practice of fundal pressure was found between doctors and nurse-midwives. Doctors reported using fundal pressure "frequently" for primigravidas' and "sometimes" for multigravidas' whereas nurse-midwives reported doing this procedure less frequently than doctors. The procedure is often performed by the care providers even though there is no evidence suggesting that it is an appropriate or safe technique to be used during second stage of labor (Simpson & Thorman, 2005).

Finally, another yet very important finding of this study was that continuous support either from caregivers or family members was not provided to mothers during labor and delivery by these care providers in India. This may be due to cultural and traditional values in India. However, the importance of continuous support either from family or care givers is supported by the evidence and needs to be addressed by the care system (Hodnett, et al., 2003).

Overall, the self-reported intrapartum care practices in this study suggest that care provided to mothers during the intrapartum phase of childbirth are based on outdated habits rather than the guidelines provided by WHO for intrapartum care. When care is based on habits and tradition rather than current best evidence published in internationally vetted guidelines, the challenges to change beliefs and outdated care practices in order to assure evidence-based care are formidable.

The opinions and self-reported care practices of maternity care providers uncovered in this survey may or may not represent the type of intrapartum care in India as a whole. Without further research, it is difficult to generalize these findings to other states in India. Changing beliefs and practice behaviors of the maternity care providers continues to be a challenging process in low resourced countries like India. Working towards this end needs an environment that is supportive of evidence-based care that requires education, information resources, and system support for practice change.

Limitations

The three primary limitations of this study must be acknowledged.

First, the results of this survey have limited generalizibility as the study was a convenience sample of maternity care providers in New Delhi and Rajasthan, two states of India. Also, the numbers of physician respondents and care providers from private hospitals was small.

Second, although the questionnaire had face validity, this tool will need refinement for use in future studies.

Third, this study is the first of its kind done in India. No other was found that examined self-reported care practices and opinions regarding the seven elements of intrapartum care including, episiotomy, labor induction, birthing position, labor pain management, childbirth support, and communicating information and instructions to mothers during labor and delivery.

Conclusions

This survey has identified a significant gap between the self reported care practices of maternity care providers in India and the guidelines provided by WHO (1999) for care in normal childbirth. This study found that routine possibly harmful interventions such as episiotomy, labor induction, administration of opioid analgesics during labor, application of fundal pressure, and non-supportive labor and delivery care are often practiced during intrapartum care phase in both government and non-government hospitals of India. These less effective interventions in routine childbirth care raise questions concerning the norm for safe and effective maternal care. There may be a number of barriers and challenges that care providers or health care decision makers need to overcome in order to transition from common practice and rituals to evidence-based childbirth care. The strong opinion of care providers, especially towards interventions like episiotomy and lithotomy position, may constitute a major barrier to change their practice behaviors

Implications for Future Practice

This study identified the lack of evidence-based intrapartum care in India. It is imperative for health care providers to understand the hierarchy of evidence and how this evidence requires care providers to change routine practices that are considered harmful and ineffective. Efforts of the maternal health programs started in India such as Child Survival and Safe Motherhood (CSSM) by the Government of India may help this effort. Initiatives such as these that aim to replace routine care with evidence-based childbirth care and improve maternal health outcomes may require integrated changes in both the health care system as well as individual perception towards evidence-based care. The concept of evidence-based care may be new for many health care providers in low- and middle-income countries such as India. However, it is necessary to disseminate the concepts and information promoting evidence-based childbirth care in order to promote safe, effective intrapartum services. The WHO Reproductive Health Library which consists of reliable and useful information derived from Cochrane systematic reviews may be of particular help to low- and middle-income countries.

Changing care practice behaviors of health professionals is not easy to achieve. A variety of strategies such as dissemination of substantial evidence-based information though journals and other printed materials as well as continuing education workshops and conferences on evidence-based care can be implemented and tested for their usefulness in changing care providers' behavior and clinical outcomes.

Implications for Future Research

This study leaves this researcher with more questions than when the study was first conceptualized. First, a more extensive survey of maternity care providers needs to be done in India in order to develop a base for identifying the extent of problems with intrapartum care practices and to help identify priorities and strategies for implementing evidence-based practice. With an improved questionnaire, replication of this study can be

52

done with larger samples across different practice sites in India. Further, new studies can be developed to identify barriers to the adoption of evidence-based childbirth care in the Indian maternity care system. Overall, more descriptive and interventional studies should be done in developing countries to improve maternal health care outcomes,

Future studies may also need to examine the relationship between different variables associated with the implementation of evidence-based childbirth care practices such as type of care providers, and type of hospitals. This may help to identify the determinants of high quality care provided in developing countries. It would also be interesting to examine the incorporation of evidence-based practice in the educational preparation of maternity care providers.

Summary

This survey examined the self-reported practices of maternity care providers, focusing on seven elements of intrapartum care including, episiotomy, labor induction, pain management during labor, birthing position, application of fundal pressure, childbirth support, and communicating information and instructions to mothers during labor. Study findings revealed significant gaps in the congruence of respondents' self-reported intrapartum care practices with the WHO guidelines for care in normal childbirth (1996). It is anticipated that childbirth care in India will benefit in the future through the application of evidence-based care. If care providers actively seek current best evidence in their clinical practice it is possible that there will be a proportionate decrease in the incidence of maternal mortality and morbidity.

REFERENCES

AHRQ (2005, May 13). Routine use of episiotomy in uncomplicated births offers no benefits to women. *Electronic News Letter, 167*, Retrieved June 10, 2006, from http://www.ahrq.gov.

Albers, L. (1998, March/April). Midwifery management of pain in labor: the CNM data group 1996. *Journal of Nurse-Midwifery, 43*(2), 77-82.

American College of Nurse-Midwives (2004). *Position Statement: Independent Midwifery Practice.* Retrieved July 12, 2006, from http://www.midwife.org.

American College of Obstetricians and Gynecologists (1999). Induction of Labor. *Washington Practice Bulletin, 10.*

Anim, S. M., Smyth, R., & Howell, C. (2005). Epidural vs non-epidural analgesia in labor. *Cochrane Database of Syatemic Reviews,* (1).

Bakshi, R. (2006). Matrnal mortality: a woman dies every 5 minutes during childbirth in India. Retrieved June 3, 2006, from http://www.unicef.org.

Baxley, E. G. (2003, May 15). Labor induction: a decade of change. *American Family Physician, 67*(10).

Bayer, A. (2004). Population Resource Center, Elective summary: maternal mortality and morbidity . Retrieved July 11, 2006, from http://www.prcdc.org.

Berg, M., Laundgren, I., Hermansson, E., & Wahlberg, V. (1996). Women's experience of the encounter with the midwife during childbirth. *Midwifery, 12,* 11-15.

Berka, R. J., Socol, M. L., & Dooley, S. L. (1999). Risk of cesarean delivery with elective induction of labor at term in nulliaparous women. *Journal of Obstetrics and Gynecology, 94,* 600-607.

Bloom, S. L., Casey, B. M., Schatter, J. I., McIntire, D. D., & Leveno, K. J. (2006). A randomized trial of coached versus uncoached maternal pushing during the second stage of labor on postpartum pelvic structure and function. *American Journal of Obstetrics and Gynecology, 194*(1), 10-13.

Blouse, A., Kinzie, B., Sanghvi, H., & Hines, K. (2004). Developing regional experts in essential maternal and newborn care: the MNH program experience. JHPIEGO.

Bodner, A. B., Bodner, K., Kimberger, O., Lozanov, P., Husslein, P., & Mayerhofer, K. (2003). Women's position during labor: influence on maternal and neonatal outcomes. *Wein Klin Wochenschr, 115*(19-20), 720-723.

Bowers, B. B. (2002). Mother's experience of labor support: exploration of qualitative research. *Journal of Obstetrics, Gynecologic, & Neonatal Nursing, 31*(6), 742-752.

Bricker, L., & Lavender, I. (2002). Parentral opioids for labor pain relief: a systematic review. *American Journal of Obstetrics & Gynecology, 186*(5), 94-109.

British Columbia Reproductive Care (1998). Obstetric Guideline 1: induction of labor.

Buhimschi, C. S., Buhimischi, I. A., Malino, A. M., Kopelman, J. N., & Cammu, H., Martens, G., Ruyssinck, G., & Ammy, J. J. (2002, February). Outcomes after elective labor induction in nulliparous women: a matched cohort study. *American Journal of Obstetrics and Gynecology, 186*(2), 240-244.

Campero, L., Gracia, C., Diaz, C., Ortiz, O., Reynosos, S., & Langer, A. (1998). "Alone, I wouldn't have known what to do": a qualitative study on social support during labor and delivery in Mexico. *Social Science and Medicine, 47*(3), 395-403.

Carroli, G., & Belizan, J. (2000). Episiotomy for vaginal birth. *Cochrane Database Systematic Review, CD000081*(2).

Caton, D., Corry, M., Frigoletto, F., Hopkins, D., & Mayberry, L. (2002). The nature and management of labor pain: executive summary. *American Journal of Obstetrics and Gynecology, 186*(5), S9.

Childbirth Connection (2006, March 9). *Evidence-based maternity care: resource directory.* Retrieved June 12, 2006, from http://www.childbirthconnection.org.

Coalition for Improving Maternity Services (CIMS) (2003). *Fact Sheet: problems and hazards of induction of labor.* Retrieved June 10, 2006, from http://www.motherfriendly.org.

Corry, M., & Rooks, J. (1999). Public education: promoting the midwifery model of care in partnership with the maternity center association. *Journal of Nurse-Midwifery, 44*(1), 47-56.

Cosner, K. R. (1996). Use of fundal pressure during second stage of labor: a pilot study. *Journal of Nurse-Midwifery, 41,* 334-337.

Crane, J. (2001). Induction of labor at term. *SOGC Clinical Practice Guideline, 107,* 1-12.

Damanhoury, H. E., Azzam, E. E., & Ibrahim, A. W. (2003). Selected practice recommendations for pregnancy and childbirth: guidelines for health care practitioners. *Association for Health and Environment Development & Health Policies and System Program,* 42.

Declercq, E. R., Sakala, C., Corry, M., Applebaum, S., & Risher, P. (2002). Listening to mothers: report of first national US survey of women's childbearing experiences. *New York, Maternity Center Association and Harris Interactive Corporation Headquarters,* 20-21.

Dickersin, K., & Manheimer, E. (1998). The Cochrane Collaboration:evaluation of health care and services using systematic reviews of the results of randomized controlled trials. *Clinical Obstetrical Gynecology, 41,* 315-331.

Dujardin, B., Boutsen, M., De Schampheleire, I., Kulker, R., Manshande, J. P., & Bailey, J. (1995). Oxytocics in developing countries. *International Journal of Obstetrics and Gynecology, 50,* 243-251.

Everett, F. M., Evans, S., Hutchinson, M., Collins, R., & Morrison, J. C. (2005). Postpartum hemorrhage after vaginal birth: an analysis of risk factors. *Southern Medical Journal, 98*(4), 419-422.

Gail, J. D. (2001). Pregnancy and childbirth tips. *Midwifery Today, Spring,* Retrieved June 14, 2006, from http://www.birthlove.com.

Goldberg, J., & Fagan, M. (2006). *Episiotomy: indications and repair.* Retrieved June 10, 2006, from http://www.femalepatient.com.

Governemnt of India (2001-2002). Annual Report. Ministry Of Health and Family Welfare.

Graham, I. D. (2005). Too many women get episiotomy during childbirth. *Birth,* Retrieved October 30, 2005, from http://www.obgyn.healthcenteronline.com.

Gulmezoglu, A. M., & Villar, J. (2002). *The WHO Reproductive Health Library.* Retrieved June 3, 2006, from http://www.globalhealth.org.

Gupta, J. K., & Nikodem, V. C. (2003). Position for women during second stage of labor. *The Cochrane Review,* (2).

Gupta, J. K., Hofmeyr, G. J., and Smyth, R. (2004). Position in second stage of labor for women without epidural anesthesia. *Cochrane Database of Systemic Review,* (1)

Haadam, K. (1998, September 30). Review of literature on advantages and disadvantages: episiotomy: only limited protection against rupture-time for revision?. *Lakartidningen (Swedish), 95*(40), 4354-4358.

Hadi, H. (2000). Labor induction: clinical guidelines. *Clinical Obstetrics Gynecology, 43,* 524-536.

Hallgren, A., Kihlgren, M., Norberg, A., & Forslin, L. (1995). Women's description of childbirth and childbirth education before and after education and birth. *Midwifery, 11*(3), 130-137.

Hartman, K., Vishwanathan, M., Palmieri, R., Gartlehner, G., Thorp, J., & Lohr, K. N. (2005, May 4). Outcomes of routine episiotomy: a systematic review. *Journal of American Medical Association, 293*(17), 2141-2148.

Hodnett, E. (1996). Nursing support for the laboring woman. *Journal of Obstetrics, Gynecologic, & Neonatal Nursing, 25,* 257-264.

Hodnett, E. D. (2002). Review: caregiver support for women during childbirth. *Cochrane Database of Systemic Review, 5*(1), 105.

Hodnett, E., Gates, S., Hofmeyr, G. J., & Sakala, C. (2003). . *Cochrane Database of Systemic Review,* (2).

Hopkins, W. G. (2000). *Quantitative research design.* Retrieved July 5, 2006, from http://www.sportsci.org.

Howarth, G. R., & Botha, D. J. (2001). Amniotomy plus intravenous oxytocin for induction of labor. Cochrane Review.

Hueston, M. D. (1996). Factors associated with the use of episiotomy during vaginal delivery. *Obstetrics and Gynecology, 87*(6), 1001-1005.

Hunter, L. P. (2002). Being with woman: a guiding concept for the care of laboring woman. *Journal of Obstetrics, Gynecologic, & Neonatal Nursing, 31*(6), 650-657.

Ip, W. Y. (2000). Relationships between partner's support during labor and maternal outcomes. *Journal of Clinical Nursing, 9,* 265-272.

Johnson, R., Newburn, M., & Macfarlane, A. (2002). Has the medicalisation of childbirth gone too far? *British Medical Journal, 324,* 892-895.

Johnson, N., Johnson, V. A., & Gupta, J. K. (1991). Maternal position during labor. *Obstetrical and Gynecological Survey, 46*(7), 428-434.

Keene, R., DiFranco, J., & Amis, D. (2005). *Care practices that support normal birth.* Retrieved June 15, 2006, from http://www.lamaze.org.

Kennel, J., Klaus, M., Mcgrrath, S., Robertson, S., & Hinkley, C. (1991). Continuous emotional support during labor in U.S. hospital. *Journal of the American Medical Association, 265*(17), 2197-2201.

Khasholian, T. K. (2005, September). Routine in facility-based maternity care: evidence from the Arab world. *BJOG: International Journal of Obstetrics and Gynaecology, 112*(9), 1270-1276.

Kitzinger, S., Green, J. M., Chalmers, B., Keirse, M., Lindstrom, K., & Hemminki, E. (2006, June). Why do women go along with this stuff? *Birth, 33*(2), 154-158.

Kline-Kaye, V., & Miller, S. D. (1990, November-December). The use of fundal pressure during the second stage of labor: a pilot study. *Journal of Obstetrics, Gynecologic, & Neonatal Nursing, 19*(6), 511-517.

Knedle-Murray, M. E., Oakley, D. J., Wheeler, J. R., & Peterson, B. A. (1993). Production process substitution in maternity care: issues of cost, quality, and outcomes by nurse-midwives and physician providers. *Medical Care Review, 50,* 80-112.

Larsson, P. G., Christensen, P., Bergman, B., & Wallstersson, G. (1991). Advantages and disadvantages of episiotomy compared with spontaneous perineal laceration. *Gynecological and Obstetric Investigation, 31,* 213-216.

Lede, R. L., Belizan, J. M., & Carroli, G. (1996). Is routine use of episiotomy justified. *American Journal of Obstetrics and Gynecology, 174,* 1399-1402.

Leeman, L., Fontaine, P., King, V., Klien, M. C., & Ratcliffe, S. (2003). The nature and management of labor pain: part II pharmacological pain relief. *American Family Physician, 68*(6), 115-122.

Lothian, J., Amis, D., & Crenshaw, J. (2005). *Care practices that support normal birth.* Retrieved June 19, 2006, from http://www.lamaze.org.

Low, L. K., Seng, J. S., Murtland, T. L., & Oakley, D. (2000). Clinician-specific episiotomy rates: impact on perineal outcomes. *Journal of Midwifery and Women's Health, 45*(2), 87-93.

MacDorman, M. F., & Singh, G. K. (1998). Midwifer care, social and medical risk factors, and birth outcomes in Unites States. *Journal of Epidemiology and Community Health, 52,* 310-317.

Maduma-Butshe, A., Dayall, A., & Garner, P. (1998). Routine episiotomy in developing countries: time to change a harmful practice. *British Medical Journal, 316,* 1179-1180.

Maslow, A. S., & Sweeney, A. L. (2000). Elective induction of labor as a risk factor for cesarean delivery among low risk women at term. *Journal of Obstetrics and Gynecology, 95,* 917-922.

McCandlish, R. (2001). Perineal trauma: prevention and treatment. *Journal of Midwifery and Women's Health, 46*(6), 396-40.

Medical Encyclopedia (2005). *Episiotomy.* Retrieved June 13, 2005, from http://www.nlm.nih.gov/medlineplus.

Merhi, Z. O., & Awonuga, A. O. (2005). The role of uterine fundal pressure in the management of the second stage of labor: a reappraisal. *Obstetrical and Gynecological Survey, 60*(9), 599-603.

Ministry of Health and Family Welfare (Government of India) (2000-2001). *Annual Report: Maternal Health Program.* Retrieved June 25, 2006, from http://www.mohfw.nic.nin/reports.

Noronha, J. A. (2004). Effectiveness of teaching on episiotomy and perineal care among primipara women of selected hospitals in Karnataka. *Nursing Journal of India,* Retrieved July 8, 2006, from www.findarticles.com.

Oxorn, F. H. (1986). Shoulder dystocia. In F. Oxorn (Ed.), *Human Labor and Birth* (5th ed.) CT: Norwalk.

Preston, R., Crosby, E. T., Kotarba, D., Dudas, H., & Elliot, R. D. (1993). Maternal positioning affects fetal heart rate changes after epidural analgesia for labour. *Canadian Journal of Anesthesia, 40,* 1136-1141.

Public Citizen's Health Research Group (1995). Encouraging the use of nurse-midwives. Washington DC: Public Citizen's Health Research Group.

Qian, X., Smith, H., Liang, H., Liang, J., & Garner, P. (2006). Evidence-informed obstetric practice during normal birth in China: trends and influence in four hospitals. *Bio Med Central Health Services Research, 6*(29).

Reime, B., Klein, M. C., Kelly, A., Duxbury, N., Saxell, L., & Liston, R. et al. (2004). Do maternity care provider groups have different attitudes towards birth. *BJOG: an International Journal of Obstetrics and Gynecology, 111,* 1388-1393.

Renfrew, M. J., Hannah, W., Albers, L., & Floyd, E. (1998). Practices that minimizes trauma to the genital tract: a systematic review of literature. *Birth, 25*(3), 143-160.

Robert, D., Vincent, J. R., & Chestnut, D. H. (1998). Epidural analgesia during labor. *American Family Physician, 58*(8).

Rodrigues, C., & Thapar, B. (2005, October 21). *FOGSI launces "Anmol Anchal" Safe Motherhood campaign in partnership with AstraZeneca India.* Retrieved June 4, 2006, from http://www.astrazenecaindia.com.

Rooks, J. P. (1999, July/August). Evidence-based practice and its application to childbirth care for low risk women. *Journal of Nurse-Midwifery, 44*(4), 355-366.

Rosen, P. (2004). Supporting women in labor: analysis of different types of care givers. *Journal of Midwifery and Women's Health, 49*(1), 24-31.

Sackette, D., Rosenberg, W., Gray, J., Haynes, R., & Richardson, W. (1996). Evidence-based medicine:what is it and what it isn't. *British Medical Journal, 71,* 312.

Shariff, A., & Singh, G. (2002). Determinants of maternal health care utilisation in India:evidence from a recent household survey. Retrieved June 10, 2006, from http://www.eldis.org.

Sharma, S. K., Sidawi, J. E., Ramin, S. M., Lucas, M. J., Leveno, K. J., & Cunningham, F. G. (1997). Cesarean delivery: a randomized trial of epidural versus patient-controlled meperidine analgesia during labor. *Anesthesiology, 87,* 487-494.

Sheiner, E., Sarid, L., Levy, A., Seidman, D. S., & Hallak, M. (2005, September). Obstetrical risk factors and outcomes of pregnancies complicated with early PPH: a population-based study. *Journal of Maternal Fetal and Neonatal Medicine, 18*(3), 149-154.

Shorten, A., Donsante, J., & Shorten, B. (2002, March). Birth position, accoucheur, and perineal outcomes: informing women about choices of childbirth. *Birth, 29*(1), 18-27.

Signorello, L. (2000). Midline episiotomy and anal incontinence: retrospective cohort study. *British Medical Journal, 320*(7227), 86-90.

Simpson, K. R., & Atterbury, J. (2003). Trends and issues in labor induction in the United States: implications for the clinical practice. *Journal of Obstetrics, Gynecology, and Neonatal Nursing, 32,* 767-779.

Simpson, K. R., & Knox, G. E. (2001). Fundal pressure during the second stage of labor. *MCN: American Journal of Maternal Child Nursing, 26,* 64-70.

Simpson, K. R., & Thorman, K. E. (2005). Obstetrics "convinience". *Journal of Perinatala and Neonatal Nursing, 19*(2), 134-144.

Smith, H., Gulmezoglu, M., & Garner, P. (2004, Januray 28-30). *Evidence-led obstetric care: WHO Geneva Report.* Retrieved June 3, 2006, from http://www.who.org.

Steer, P. (1999). *Labor: an overview* (1 ed.). London: WB Saunders.

Stetler, C. (1999). Clinical Scholarship exemplars: the bay state medical center. *Clinical Scholarship White Paper: Sigma Theta Tau International, 1*(1), 15-16.

Summers, L. (1997). Cervical ripening and labor induction. *Journal of Nurse-Midwifery, 42*(2), 71-85.

Surg, V. (2005). Maternal Mortality: Indian Scenario. *MJAFI, 61,* 214-215. Retrieved June 22, 2006, from http://www.medind.nic.in

Thornton, P. (n.d). Labor induction: "can you induce my labor"? sure you can, but may be you shouldn't. *Expectant Mother's Guide.* Retrieved June 14, 2006, from http://www.expectantmothersguide.com.

Tillett, J. (2005, April/June). Obstetrics rituals: is practice supported by evidence. *Journal of Perinatal & Neonatal Nursing,* 91-93.

UNFPA . *Saving Mother's Lives: The Challenge Continues.* Retrieved July 5, 2006, from http://www.unfpa.org.

UNFPA (2006, May 5, 2006). World needs midwives more than ever to keep more women, babies alive, say global health actors on International Midwives Day. *Press Release.* Retrieved July 11, 2006, from http://www.unfpa.org.

Usta, I. M., Mercer, B. M., & Sibai, B. M. (1999). Current obstetrical practice and umbilical cord prolapse. *American Journal of Perinatology, 16,* 479-484.

Vangeenderhuysen, C., & Souidi, A. (2002). Uterine rupture of pregnant uterus: study of a continuous series of 63 cases at the referral maternity of Niamey (Niger). *Med Trop (Mars), 62,* 615-616.

Volmink, J., Murphy, C., & Woldehannas, S. (2002, May). Towards an evidence-based approach to decision making: making childbirth safer through promoting evidence-based care. Retrieved June 3, 2006, from http://www.globalhealth.org.

WHO (2003). Pregnancy, childbirth, postpartum, and newborn care: a guide fro essential practice. Retrieved June 10, 2006, from http://www.who.org.

Wick, L., Mikki, N., Giacaman, R., & Abdul-Rahim, H. (2005, January 18). Childbirth in Palestine. *International Journal of Gynecology and Obstetrics, 89,* 174-178.
Wikepedia Encyclopedia (2006, May 30). *Qualitative research.* Retrieved June 7, 2006, from http://www.en.wikepedia.org.

Williams, F. L., Florey, C. D., Mires, G. J., & Ogston, S. A. (1998). Episiotomy and perineal tears in low risk U.K. primigravida. *Journal of Public Health Medicine, 20*(4), 422-427.

World Health Organization (1999). Care in normal birth: a practical guide. The World Health Organization Report.

World Health Organization (2000). Making Pregnancy Safer: report by the secretariat. Geneva:WHO.

World Health Organization (2005). Clinical Practice Guidelines. The WHO Reproductive Health Library, 8.

APPENDICES

APPENDIX A

SURVEY QUESTIONNAIRE

Dear participant

Thank you for participating and taking time to fill out this survey. The purpose of the survey is to examine the self-reported practice activities of maternity care providers during intranatal period. Your participation is voluntary. You may refuse to participate in this survey at anytime. There are no known risks involved. You may request a summary of my findings via e-mail at rko2@unh.edu. I am conducting this study to pursue my master's in nursing degree at University of New Hampshire.

Thank you for your cooperation

Rizwana
Graduate student
University of New Hampshire

Name of the hospital/Institution: _____

1. What *position* do you have?

    Doctor   ☐   Nurse-midwife   ☐

               1   2

2. How many *years of experience* do you have in Labor and Delivery?

_____

3. At your place of work normal birth are *attended* commonly by:

Doctors'   ☐   1

Nurse Midwives   ☐   2

Both   ☐   3

4. Do you have **written policies** concerning normal birth?

Yes ☐ 1

No ☐ 2

Don't know ☐ 3

5. If yes, please specify, **what standard** they are based on?

_____

_____

_____

6. Do doctors and midwives use the **same procedures** for normal birth?

Yes ☐   No ☐   Don't know ☐
  1   2   3

7. If no, please specify the reason?

_____

_____

_____

_____

_____

_____

Please answer the following questions according to your **practice?**

Episiotomies **should be** performed:

	Strongly agree	Agree	Disagree	Strongly disagree
8. For nearly all deliveries	☐	☐	☐	☐
9. Nearly all primigravidas'	☐	☐	☐	☐
10. Anyone who would tear	☐	☐	☐	☐
	1	2	3	4

11. In your practice how *often* do you perform episiotomies?

	always	frequently	sometimes	rarely	never
Primigravida	☐	☐	☐	☐	☐
Multigravida	☐	☐	☐	☐	☐
	1	2	3	4	5

12. When deciding on doing an episiotomy do you *consider mothers' preference* for doing it?

Yes ☐   No ☐   Unable to answer ☐

1   2   3

13. If no, please specify why you *do not consider* the mothers' preference?

_____

_____

_____

_____

_____

14. From your own practice experience, what do you think what causes more *discomfort* to mother?

Episiotomy ☐   Perineal laceration of same depth ☐   Both equally ☐

1   2   3

15. From your own practice experience which results in higher rate of *vulval- hematoma?*

Episiotomy ☐   Perineal laceration of same depth ☐   Both equally ☐

1   2   3

16. In your views what are the benefits or drawbacks of *episiotomy vs. Laceration* of same depth?

_____

_____

_____

17. What *methods of pain relief* do you use during the first stage of labor?

a. Pharmacological: Yes ☐   No ☐

                          1   2

18. If yes, please specify *what drugs* you may use for pain relief during the first stage of labor?

_____

_____

_____

_____

b. Non-Pharmacological: Yes ☐   No ☐

                                 1   2

19. If yes, please *list* down all the methods you may use?

_____

_____

_____

20. From your own practice experience, what percentage of women receive the following *pain relief* measures?

	Pharmacological	Non-pharmacological
Primigravida	_____	_____
Multigravida	_____	_____

21. In your institution, how *often* does the mother deliver in the following position?

	always	frequently	sometimes	rarely	never
a. Lithotomy	☐	☐	☐	☐	☐
b. Semi-sitting	☐	☐	☐	☐	☐
c. Lateral	☐	☐	☐	☐	☐
d. Upright	☐	☐	☐	☐	☐
e. Squatting	☐	☐	☐	☐	☐
	1	2	3	4	5

22. What do you think is the *preferred position* for the mother to deliver?

_____

23. Please specify, *why* do you prefer the above mentioned position for the mother to deliver?

_____

_____

_____

_____

_____

24. Do you use *routinely* induce labor?   Yes ☐   No ☐
                                              1   2

25. If yes, specify *what method* you may use to induce labor?

Drugs ☐   AROM ☐   Both ☐

        1   2   3

26. If yes, please specify what drugs you may administer to induce the labor?

_____

_____

_____

27. From your own practice experience, what percentage of low risk women undergoes labor induction?

	By drugs	By AROM
Primigravida	_____	_____
Multigravida	_____	_____

28. From your own practice experience, how **frequently** do the mothers receive fundal pressure to assist in normal delivery?

	always	frequently	sometimes	rarely	never
Primigravida	☐	☐	☐	☐	☐
Multigravida	☐	☐	☐	☐	☐
	1	2	3	4	5

29. How **often** do you provide routine information and explanation to the mothers during labor & delivery?

always ☐   frequently ☐   sometimes ☐   rarely ☐   never ☐
  1   2   3   4   5

30. Please **list** down the information you provide to the mother during labor & delivery?

1st stage:-

_____

_____

_____

_____

_____

_____

2nd stage:-

_____

_____

_____

_____

_____

_____

31. Is the mother permitted to have a **support person** during labor & delivery?

Yes ☐   No ☐
     1   2

32. If yes, please specify **who**?

_____

33. If yes, please specify if the **support person constantly** remains with the mother during labor and delivery?

_____

_____

34. Is there anything else you would like to add, please do so in space provided here:

_____

_____

_____

_____

_____

_____

Thank you for participating!!!!!!!!!!

68

INFORMED CONSENT

Dear participant,

I am a graduate student enrolled in the Master of Science in Clinical Leadership program at the University of New Hampshire (New Hampshire, U.S).I am conducting a study related to "Evidence based obstetrical practices in India". Enclosed is a survey related to attitudes and practices of maternity care providers during intrapartum management among maternity care providers".

Participation in the survey is entirely voluntary. There are no known risks involved in the study. If you choose to participate you may benefit by understanding of maternal care knowledge and practices.

I would like to ask you to complete and return the survey by 1st week of January 2006 to the given address via mail or it can be given directly to the investigator during follow up visits. The questionnaire asks for no identification information, only aggregate data will be reported. All results will be kept confidential.

Completing the survey represents your consent to participate

If you have any questions or concerns please feel free to contact me or my faculty advisor at the address given below. For more information regarding your rights as a research subject contact *Research Conduct and Compliance Services staff*: Julie Simpson, Manger, at julie.simpson@unh.edu or 001-603-862-2003, or Kathleen Stilwell, Assistant, at Kathy.stilwell@unh.edu or 001-603-862-3536. Additional materials are available at http://www.unh.eu/osr/compliance/irb.html

Contacts:

Investigator

Ms. Rizwana
Address: c/o Mr. M.I. Ansari
J-4 Jamia Hamdard
New Delhi, 110062 (India)
Home Phone: 55826588
email: rko2@unh.edu

Advisor

Dr. Gene Harkless
Associate Professor
Dept.of Nursing
UNH, Durham
New Hampshire
03824 (United States)
Office ph# 001-603-862-2285
email: gene.harkless@unh.edu

_____   _____

Signature of investigator   Date

APPENDIX C

UNH INSTITUTIONAL REVIEW BOARD APPROVAL

APPENDIX   C

UNIVERSITY *of* NEW HAMPSHIRE

November 8, 2005

Rizwana
Nursing, Hewitt Hall
175 Forest Park
Durham, NH 03824

IRB #:   3547
Study: Intrapartum Care Practices in India: A Survey of Maternity Care
                    Providers
Approval Date: 11/02/2005

The Institutional Review Board for the Protection of Human Subjects in Research (IRB) has reviewed and approved the protocol for your study as Exempt as described in Title 45, Code of Federal Regulations (CFR), Part 46, Subsection 101(b). Approval is granted to conduct your study as described in your protocol.

Researchers who conduct studies involving human subjects have responsibilities as outlined in the attached document, *Responsibilities of Directors of Research Studies Involving Human Subjects*.   (This   document   is   also   available   at http://www.unh.edu/osr/compliance/irb.html.) Please read this document carefully before commencing your work involving human subjects.

Upon completion of your study, please complete the enclosed pink Exempt Study Final Report form and return it to this office along with a report of your findings.

If you have questions or concerns about your study or this approval, please feel free to contact me at 603-862-2003 or Julie.simpson@unh.edu. Please refer to the IRB # above in all correspondence related to this study. The IRB wishes you success with your research.

For the IRB,

Julie F. Simpson
Manager

cc: File
       Gene Harkless

**Research Conduct and Compliance Services, Office of Sponsored Research, Service
Building, 51 College Road, Durham, NH 03824-3585 * Fax: 603-862-3564**

64

www.ingramcontent.com/pod-product-compliance
Lightning Source LLC
Chambersburg PA
CBHW072155020426
42334CB00018B/2019

* 9 7 8 3 6 3 9 0 1 4 5 1 8 *